Copycat Recipes

Complete Copycat cookbook to prepare the recipes of your favorite restaurants at home. Step by step guide with cooking techniques and easy-to-prepare recipes

Table of contents

INTRODUCTION 9

- Tomatoes stuffed with tuna 19
- Copycat Krispy Kreme Donuts Glazed 21
- Roasted Pumpkin Seeds 27
- Homemade Spicy Beef Jerky 31
- Caviar Deviled Eggs 37
- Thai Chicken Coconut Milk Soup 40
- Corn Cream Recipe 46
- Zucchini cream 50
- Pumpkin cream soup 54
- Pumpkin cream with edible mushrooms 59
- Salmon gravlax 63
- Salmon recipe with grilled eggplants and chickpea croutons .. 68
- Zucchini noodles with shrimp 74
- Salmon piccata with lemon sauce 76
- Avocado and fish cake 80

COPYCAT RECIPES

© Copyright 2020 Master American Kitchen all rights reserved

This document is geared towards providing exact and reliable information with regard to the topic and issue covered. The publication is sold with the idea that the publisher is not required to render accounting, officially permitted, or otherwise qualified services. If advice is necessary, legal or professional, a practiced individual in the profession should be ordered.

From a Declaration of Principles which was accepted and approved equally by a Committee of the American Bar Association and a Committee of Publishers and Associations.

In no way is it legal to reproduce, duplicate, or transmit any part of this document in either electronic means or in printed format. Recording of this publication is strictly prohibited, and any storage of this document is not allowed unless with written permission from the publisher. All rights reserved.

The information provided herein is stated to be truthful and consistent, in that any liability, in terms of inattention or otherwise, by any usage or abuse of any policies, processes, or directions contained within is the solitary and utter responsibility of the recipient reader. Under no circumstances will any legal responsibility or blame be held against the publisher for any reparation, damages, or monetary loss due to the information herein, either directly or indirectly.

INTRODUCTION

Copycat recipes really please the home cook! Whether you're preparing food for your family or having fun with your friends or business colleagues, a copycat recipe will ensure that you're serving an unforgettable meal that brings joy to your friends and family.

Famous copycat recipe is the recipe that you can replicate and cook in your own home from your favorite restaurants. What's the popular recipe for copycat? The chefs usually pick up a meal at a restaurant and figure out what ingredients make the dish so delicious. The ingredients used the exact measurement and how long cooking takes. These have been translated into a new variety and collected as a recipe book.

You can now bring the kitchen of your favorite restaurant to your own home with the help of the famous copycat recipe and be the chef to cook hundreds of your favorite gourmet recipes. Say goodbye to long hours of waiting in a restaurant just to sit down and most of all say goodbye to paying too much in an expensive restaurant each time you visit.

Cooking at home can take a long time and create chaos that you need to clear up, but once you've finished and tried a particular dish, you're going to be shocked and proud that you've created a very popular, delicious dish and become a professional chef. Surprise you every day, because everything is in your hands with the famous copy of the copycat

Famous copycat recipes are the recipes in your favorite restaurants at home that you can mimic and prepare. What's the famous imitator recipe? In a restaurant, the chefs usually eat to figure out what ingredients make the food so delicious. The ingredients used the exact measure and the length of time needed for cooking. These have been translated into a new variety and published as a book for the recipe. You can now add the kitchen of your favorite restaurant to your home with the aid of the popular copycat recipe and, as a chef, prepare hundreds of your favorite gourmet recipes. Say goodbye to a restaurant's long waiting to take a seat, and in particular say goodbye to paying too much every time you visit an expensive restaurant.

Cooking at home can take a long time and create chaos that you need to clear up, but once you've finished and tried a particular dish, you're going to be shocked and proud that you've created a very popular, delicious dish and become a professional chef. Surprise you every day because everything is in your hands with the famous copy of the copycat.

Reasons Copycat Recipes Are Better Than Eating at Restaurants

1. Health

It's great to make copycat recipes at home. They give you the exact ingredients, but as you see fit, you can modify them. Whether you want to taste different food or add your own vegetables, it doesn't matter.

You can also add low-fat ingredients or remove allergic ingredients. There are endless possibilities. You are in complete control. Like the original dishes, how do you learn these recipes taste?

2. Quality

A team of professional chefs will create these recipes. So ensure that you get the exact ingredients and measures so make your favorite dish, they are continuously sampled. Of course, recipes that are said to be imitations of popular restaurants can be searched online. Yeah, it's safe. And there's a reason they're safe. They're not true recipes for copycat. They're just not even near. I tried several of them, and to be honest, they weren't just there, they weren't good either. I'm going to show you how to get the true copycat recipes and how to get your freedom back.

3. Freedom

Do you know how much time you spend dining out and how much freedom? Will you at midnight get your favorite food? While watching your favorite series, will you eat your favorite food? For starters, you're driving to the restaurant, waiting for a table, waiting for an appetizer, waiting for a meal, waiting for a dessert, and you guessed it, waiting to get your bill paid. So how long are you waiting for? Two hours, three more hours? Take your free time and prepare your favorite home-made dishes. Use these recipes of copycat to prepare your favorite dish when and how you want it.

4. Variety

There are copycat recipes for almost every popular restaurant. Here are some of the restaurants to give you an idea: Outback Steakhouse, Apple Bees, Olive Garden, Red Lobster, Chilies, Starbucks, PF Changs, KFC, Wendys and the list goes on and on. Does one of these recipes offer a low-fat or organic variant?

Tomatoes stuffed with tuna

Ingredients

- 2 cans of water or natural tuna
- 4 medium tomatoes
- 1 large cup of white or brown rice
- Mayonnaise c / n
- Green olives c / n
- Peas or capers c / n
- 2 carrots
- Salt c / n

Direction

- Place plenty of water in a pot and bring it to the fire. When it boils, pour the rice. Stir with a wooden spoon so that it does not stick and cook for 20 minutes or until it is soft. Remove, drain immediately and reserve in the fridge.

- Peel the carrots and cut them into small cubes. Cook in a pot with water until they soften. Drain and place in a bowl.
- Add the rice, the two cans of drained tuna, the peas or capers (cooked) and the mayonnaise to taste.
- Mix everything very well and room to taste.
- Wash the tomatoes very well and smoke them with the help of a knife and a spoon.
- If you want to take advantage of what you have taken to the tomato, cut it into small cubes and mix it with the rice or reserve it for another recipe.
- Fill the tomatoes with the rice and the tuna. Garnish with some mayonnaise in the center and a green olive.

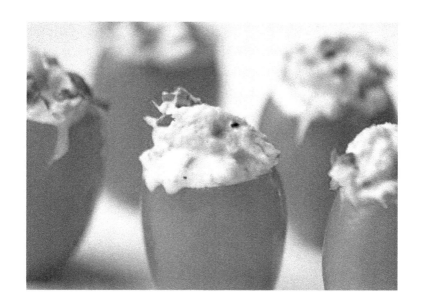

Copycat Krispy Kreme Donuts Glazed

Ingredient

Donuts

- 2 1/4 teaspoons active dry yeast
- 1/2 cup warm water, 110 degrees
- 1/4 cup granulated sugar, divided
- 1/4 cup evaporated milk, heated to 110 degrees
- 1/2 teaspoon salt
- 1/4 cup shortening, at room temperature
- 1 large egg
- 1 egg yolk
- 1/2 teaspoon vanilla extract
- 2 1/2 cups all-purpose flour, then more as needed
- 3 - 4 cups of shortening, for frying

Glaze

- 2 tablespoons unsalted butter, melted
- 1 1/3 cups of powdered sugar
- 1 pinch of salt
- 2 teaspoons evaporated milk
- 1/2 teaspoon vanilla extract
- 3 - 4 teaspoons hot water

direction

- In the bowl of an electric mixer, mix the yeast, warm water and 1/2 teaspoon of sugar. Let stand 5 to 10 minutes. Add the evaporated milk, the remaining granulated sugar (3 tablespoons + 2 1/2 teaspoons), salt, 1/4 cup butter, egg, egg yolk, and vanilla. Add half the flour and adjust the blender with the whisk and mix until smooth. Change the blender to the hook attachment, slowly add the remaining flour and knead at low speed until it is smooth and elastic for approximately 4 to 5 minutes, adding additional flour as needed (I only added approximately 2 tablespoons more. You should not need much more, you want the dough should be slightly sticky and sticky, but should not adhere to the tip of the clean finger). Transfer the dough to a lightly greased bowl,

- Knock the dough down and roll in a uniform layer on a floured surface with a thickness of less than 1/2 inch. Donut-shaped cut with a donut cutter or two round circular cutters (one large and one small for holes). Cover and let rise until doubled, approximately 30 to 40 minutes.
- Reduce heat in a Dutch cast-iron oven to 360 degrees (do not move away from oil during preheating and do not allow it to exceed 375 degrees, remove from heat and reduce heat as necessary).

Meanwhile, prepare the glaze by mixing all the glaze ingredients in a shallow dish (do not add too much water, you will dip hot donuts in the glaze so you don't want it to be liquid, quite thick is good). Carefully transfer the donuts to the oil (it could fry 3 at a time) and fry until golden brown on the bottom, then use a wooden stick, turn to the opposite side and fry the opposite side until golden brown. Transfer to a wire rack and let it cool for 1 to 2 minutes, then immerse the upper half in the enamel while it is still hot and return to the wire rack and allow the enamel to set at room temperature. Better served warm. Once cold, reheat in the microwave for 5 to 10 seconds if desired.
- Recipe Source: Classy Kitchen

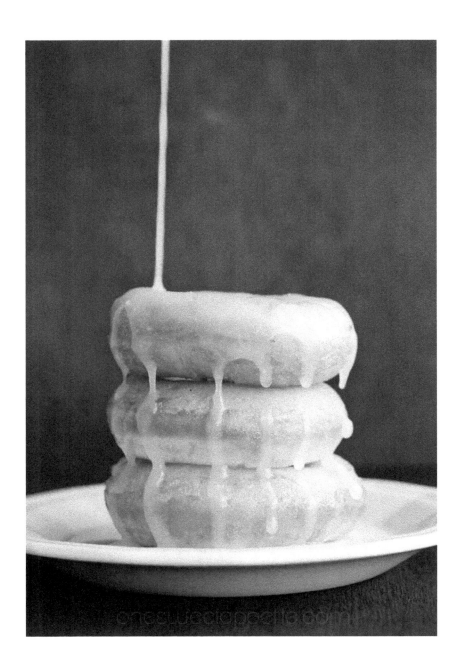

Roasted Pumpkin Seeds

Ingredients
- 1 pumpkin
- Olive oil
- Salt
- Spices to taste (salt and pepper, paprika, cinnamon and sugar, curry, etc.)

Instructions
- We preheat the oven to 200 ° C (400 ° F)
- Remove the pumpkin seeds
- We remove the pulp from the seeds and wash them in cold water
- In a pot, we will boil the seeds, use 2 cups of water for every 1/2 cup of seeds
- Add a teaspoon of salt for each cup of water and let them simmer for 10 minutes
- We remove the water and dry
- On a baking sheet, we put olive oil

- We place the seeds on top of the oil and season them to our liking
- Bake for 25 to 40 minutes (until golden brown and crispy)
- I eat them as a whole - although there are people who prefer to only eat the small seed inside.

Nutrition

Calories: 72kcal Carbohydrates: 1 g Protein: 3 g Fat: 6 g Saturated fat: 1 g Sodium: 255 mg Potassium: 86 mg Fiber: 0 g Sugar: 0 g Vitamin A: 45IU Vitamin C: 0.2 mg Calcium: 5 mg Iron: 0.9 mg

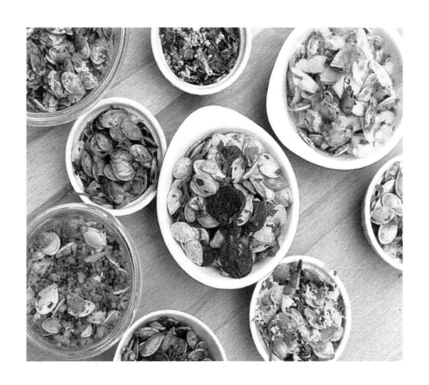

Homemade Spicy Beef Jerky

Ingredients

- 1 kg of roulades from a butcher or another lean beef, 4-5mm thick slices
- 100 ml soy sauce *
- 150 ml organic apple cider vinegar
- 1 tbsp Sambal Oelek *
- Salt pepper
- 1 pinch of stevia *

Preparation

- Mix the ingredients for the marinade thoroughly.
- Remove any fat from the meat and cut it into the desired portions.
- Put the meat and marinade alternately in a food bag.
- If possible, squeeze the air out of the bag and seal it.

- Leave to marinate in the fridge for twelve to 24 hours.
- Drain, dab thoroughly with kitchen paper.
- Allow drying on a grid at around 50 degrees in the oven (leave the air and a small gap open) or in the automatic dehydrator for about 8-10 hours.

Nutritional information

Serving: 1 total | Calories: 860 kcal | Carbohydrates: 95 g | Protein: 48 g | Fat: 32 g

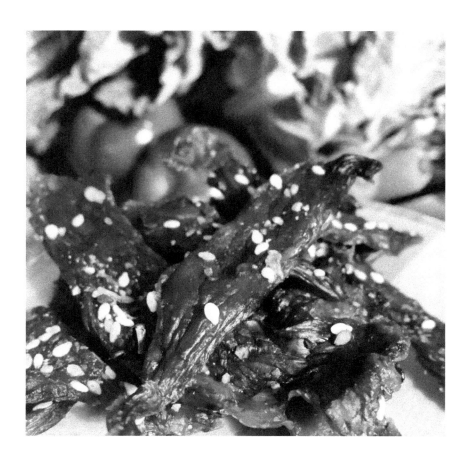

Caviar Deviled Eggs

The recipe for stuffed eggs with Caviar is one of the easiest recipes that can be made, but also one of the richest. Who has not eaten them stuffed with tuna at any time? Well, in this case we will prepare them with sturgeon roe. The truth today I do not know anyone who does not like, despite the simplicity of the recipe.

Ingredients

- 4 eggs
- 2 tablespoons fresh cream
- 1/2 teaspoon paprika
- a pinch of salt
- 30 g of Caviar
- 1 sprig of fresh dill

Preparation

- Boil the eggs. Fill a saucepan with water, introduce the eggs and put them in the

stove. When it starts to boil, count 5 minutes and remove from heat.
- Cool them with water, and then remove them carefully, to preserve the bright appearance of the egg.
- Take a knife and cut the eggs in half. With a spoon, remove the yolk from the inside, taking care not to break the white part. Place all the bears in a separate container.
- To the yolks, add the fresh cream and paprika. Mix well until a thin smooth cream is made.
- On a plate, place the halves of the eggs. Fill the interior with the mixture you have created with the yolks. Cover with the sturgeon eggs that you have chosen on top of the mixture.
- To decorate, sprinkle some paprika to give it a touch of color. Then put some dill

leaves on the mixture and next to the caviar.

Nutrition

Calories: 106kcal Carbohydrate: 3 g Protein: 7 g Fat: 6 g Saturated fat: 2 g Cholesterol: 215 mg Sodium: 301 mg Potassium: 80 mg Fiber: 0 g Sugar: 1 g Vitamin A: 335IU Calcium: 39 mg Iron: 1.2 mg

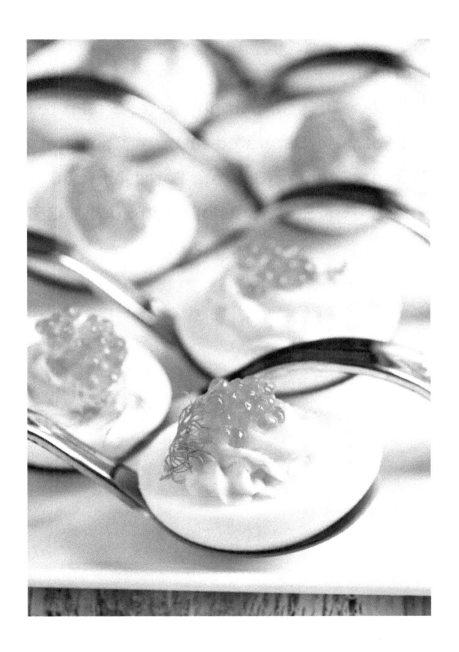

Thai Chicken Coconut Milk Soup

Ingredients

- 1 lemongrass stalk
- 6 cups chicken broth
- 2 chicken breasts
- 4 kaffir lime leaves
- 2 fresh and chopped red chili peppers
- 1 piece of ginger the size of a thumb and grated
- 400 ml of good quality coconut milk
- 2 tablespoons fish fumet (or more to taste)
- 2 tablespoons lemon juice
- A handful of fresh basil leaves
- A handful of fresh coriander leaves
- OPTIONAL: Sliced pepper (or cherry tomatoes)
- OPTIONAL: 1 teaspoon brown sugar
- OPTIONAL: wheat or rice noodles

Direction
- Cut and chop the bottom of the lemongrass stalk. Keep the upper stem for later.
- Put the chicken stock in a large pot and bring to medium-high heat. If you have leftover chicken or turkey bones, add them too. Let it boil.
- Add sliced skinless chicken breasts and mushrooms.
- Next, add the lemongrass, the upper stem, the kaffir lime leaves, and the fresh chiles.
- Boil for 5 to 8 minutes or until the chicken is well cooked. Lower the heat to medium.
- Add ginger, 200 ml of coconut milk, fish sauce and additional vegetables (if you use). Stir well and simmer for a couple of minutes. Lower the heat.
- Add the lime juice and stir.

- Do tastes test. Find the balance between acidic, spicy, salty and sweet flavors. Start with salinity; add more fish fumet if the soup is not salty or tasty enough, one tablespoon at a time. If it is very bitter, add brown sugar. If the soup is very spicy or if you want it to be creamier, add more coconut milk. If it is not spicy enough, add more chiles.
- Serve Thai chicken soup in serving bowls. Sprinkle some fresh cilantro, chives, and basil over each bowl.
- If you are going to serve the soup with noodles, it is better to prepare them separately; otherwise, the soup will become thick due to the starch of the noodles.

Nutrition

Calories 357 Calories from Fat 63% Protein 29g Fat 25g Sat fat 19g Carbohydrate 7.2g Fiber 0.5g Sodium 484mg Cholesterol 79mg

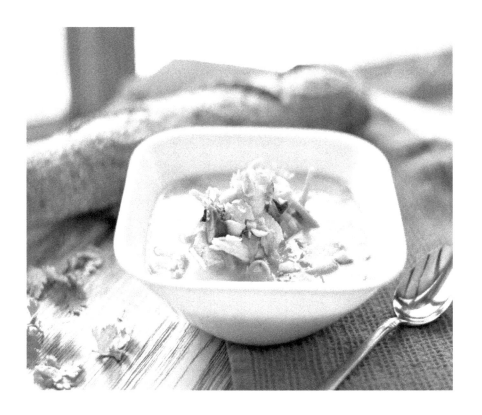

Corn Cream Recipe

Ingredients

- 1 ear of corn
- 1 yellow pepper
- 1 onion
- 1 tablespoon butter
- 1 splash of cream
- Vegetable soup
- 1 dash of extra virgin olive oil

Direction

- Place the butter in a pan and brown the previously peeled and finely chopped onion.
- When the onion is transparent, add the yellow pepper cut into small cubes along with the corn and a drizzle of extra virgin olive oil.

- When the vegetables are golden brown, cover with the vegetable stock.
- Crush the preparation with a splash of cream or milk cream and serve the hot corn cream. Garnish with corn kernels and chopped parsley.

Nutritional information

Per serving: 253 calories; 16.5 g fat; 24.8 g carbohydrates; 5.1 g protein; 54 mg cholesterol; 373 mg sodium.

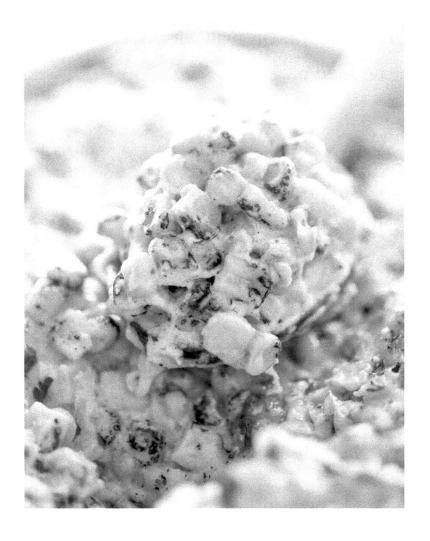

Zucchini cream

Ingredients

- 3 medium zucchini
- 1 onion
- 1 large potato
- ½ leek
- 200ml of water
- 100ml of cream or liquid cream
- 30ml olive oil
- 1 tablet of chicken broth

Direction

- Wash all the vegetables.
- Chop the zucchini, leek, onion, and potato into small cubes.
- Heat the olive oil in a pot and sauté the onion and the leek.

- Add the zucchini and potato and sauté for five minutes or until the zucchini takes a little color.
- Add a tablet of broth and a glass of water and cook for 20 more minutes.
- Remove from heat and mash the vegetables with the blender until you get a creamy texture. Finally, add the cream and mix. Season with salt and ground black pepper

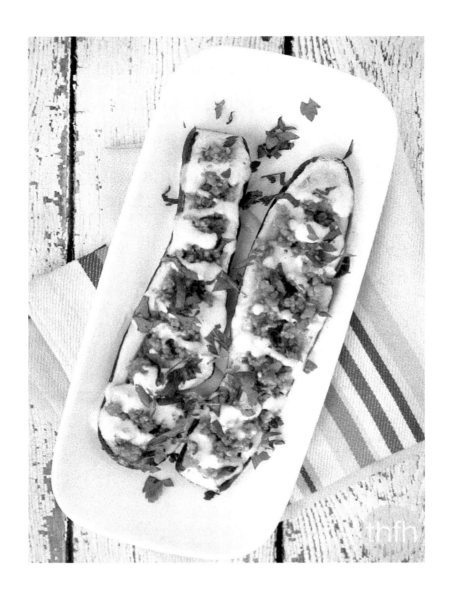

Pumpkin cream soup

Ingredients

- 1 pumpkin of 1 kilo or pumpkin
- ¼ onion
- 2 butter spoons
- 2 tablespoons flour
- 2 tablespoons olive oil
- ¾ cups of cream or milk cream
- Toasted bread
- 2 cups chicken broth
- A handful of chopped fresh parsley
- Salt and ground black pepper

Direction

- Cut the squash into pieces and remove the seeds and fibers by scraping with a spoon.
- Place the pumpkin in a microwave-safe container and cook for 10 minutes. Remove and if it is soft, remove the peel

and place the pulp in a blender together with the chicken broth. Blend until it is completely ground. If you do not have a microwave oven, do not worry, because you can cook the pumpkin cut into pieces in water until it is very tender and even make it baked.
- Put the butter and oil in a pot and bring it to the fire. When hot add the peeled and finely chopped onion and cook until transparent.
- Add the flour and mix quickly. Cook for a few minutes until golden brown.
- Pour the liquid pumpkin and cook over medium heat for 10 minutes, stirring occasionally.
- Season with salt and ground black pepper to taste and add the cream or milk cream. Cook for a couple of minutes. If the

pumpkin cream soup is very thick, you can add water or chicken broth.
- Serve the pumpkin cream soup on a soup plate or in bowls and decorate with pieces of toast, parsley and pumpkin seeds

Nutrition Facts

Per Serving: 322 calories; 25.4 g fat; 20.2 g carbohydrates; 5.1 g protein; 83 mg cholesterol; 1313 mg sodium.

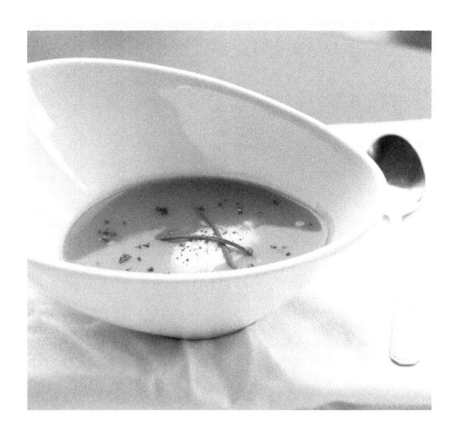

Pumpkin cream with edible mushrooms

Ingredients

- 1 large pumpkin
- 500c.c. chicken broth
- 350g edible mushrooms
- 100g grated Parmesan cheese
- 1 onion
- 2 cloves of garlic
- A splash of liquid cream
- Salt and nutmeg c / n
- Olive oil c / n

Direction

- Clean the pumpkin and peel it.
- Cut it in half and pass a peeled garlic clove so that the pulp is impregnated with the flavor.

- Place on a tray; pour a little olive oil over the pumpkin and bake for 60 minutes at 250 ° C.
- After this period of time, place the baked pumpkin in a saucepan with the chicken stock and the peeled onion; cook for 20 minutes.
- When the squash is soft, crush everything in a blender.
- Add some grated Parmesan cheese and continue crushing.
- Place some olive oil with the remaining garlic clove peeled and chopped and sauté the rolled edible mushrooms. When the mushrooms are cooked, reserve them.
- Serve the pumpkin cream in soup dishes or clay casseroles with a little grated Parmesan cheese, salt and nutmeg, cream and mushrooms.

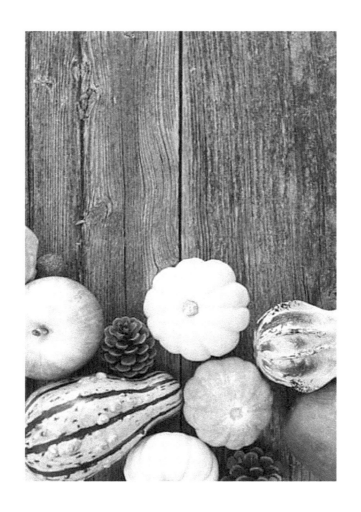

Salmon gravlax

Ingredients

- 2 salmon fillets of 1 kilo each, without skin
- ¼ cup vodka
- 1/3 cup fine sea salt
- 1/3 cup sugar
- 1 tablespoon ground black pepper
- ¼ cup chopped dill

Direction

- Gather the ingredients of salmon gravlax.
- Rinse the salmon fillets and dry them well.
- Use pliers or pliers to remove the spines if necessary.
- Sprinkle the salmon evenly with the vodka.
- In a small bowl combine sugar, fine sea salt and ground black pepper.

- Divide the mixture into three equal parts inside the bowl.
- Put half of the one-third of the curing mixture on a rimmed baking sheet.
- Place a skinless salmon fillet on the mixture and spread a third in the mixture on the fillet.
- Spread the other half of the third over the second steak and sprinkle both with chopped dill.
- Place the second fillet on the first and sprinkle the remaining curing mixture on the skin of the upper salmon.
- Cover the tray with foil and place a wooden board on the covered fish. Cover with a heavy pot and bring it to the refrigerator for at least 12 hours.
- Remove from the refrigerator and discard the accumulated liquid in the tray. Bring

the salmon back in the refrigerator for 12 hours.
- Its fish is already cured and you can serve it, but it will continue to benefit from another 12 to 24 hours of refrigeration.Nutritional Guidelines (per serving)
- 238 Calories
- 12g Fat
- 3g Carbs
- 27g Protein

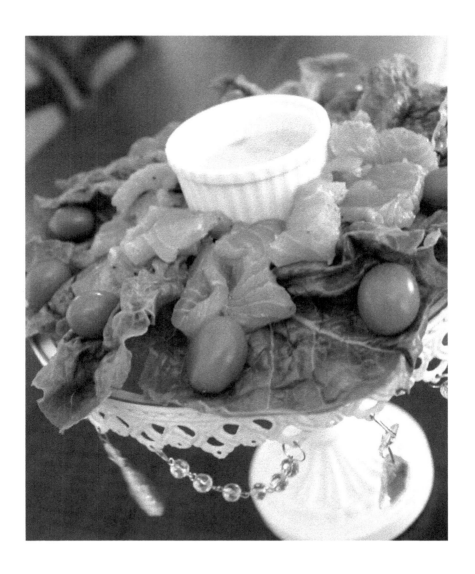

Salmon recipe with grilled eggplants and chickpea croutons

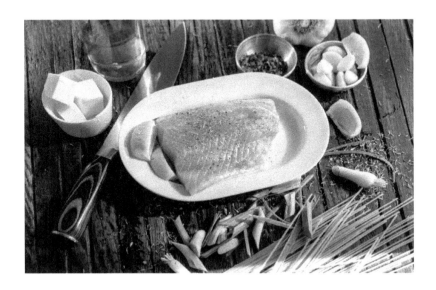

Ingredients

- 3 tablespoon plus 1 teaspoon olive oil
- 1 onion, finely chopped
- 2 cloves garlic, minced
- 1 cup chickpea flour
- 1 tablespoon lemon zest
- 2 teaspoons lemon juice
- 2 medium eggplants

- 600 g of skinless salmon fillet, cut into 4 pieces
- ¼ cup plain nonfat yogurt
- 1 cup mint leaves
- 2 tablespoons chopped chives

Direction

- Cover mold with parchment paper.
- Heat a tablespoon of oil in a pan and bring to medium heat. Add one of the garlic and chopped onion and room to taste, stirring constantly, until everything is tender,
- Add two cups of water and when it boils, add the chickpea flour and beat vigorously, out of the heat until there are almost no lumps left.
- Bring the mixture to the lemon zest food processor and puree, gradually adding a tablespoon of oil until it is completely smooth,

- Transfer to the mold and cover with another piece of parchment paper. Put a mole up and press with a heavy object. Refrigerate until firm.
- Heat the grill to medium-high. Cut the chickpea mixture into 1.5 cm cubes. Heat a teaspoon of oil in a small pan and cook the chickpea croutons until golden brown, turning occasionally. Transfer to a paper towel to remove excess oil.
- Slice the eggplant lengthwise and brush the eggplant slices with the rest of the oil. Sauté with salt and handle until tender, 3 to 4 minutes.
- Season the salmon with salt and ground black pepper and add to the grill together with the eggplant and cook for 5 minutes on each side.
- In a small bowl, mix yogurt, chopped garlic clove, lemon juice, and salt. Sprinkle

the yogurt sauce over the eggplants and accompany with chickpea croutons, chopped chives, and mint. Serve with grilled salmon.

Zucchini noodles with shrimp

Ingredients

- 750 g of peeled and deveined shrimp
- ¼ cup dry vermouth
- 1/3 cup lemon juice
- 5 zucchini
- 2 tablespoons unsalted butter
- 2 tablespoons chopped fresh parsley
- 2 tablespoons olive oil
- 2 tablespoons minced garlic
- 3 teaspoons lemon peel
- ½ teaspoon red pepper
- Parmesan cheese c / n
- Salt and ground black pepper to taste

Direction

- Create a zucchini zoodles with a spiralizer.
- Season the shrimp with salt and ground black pepper.

- Heat the butter and oil together in a pan over medium heat. Once the butter melts, add the garlic and shrimp.
- Cook the shrimp for two to three minutes, until they are pink and cooked. Remove and reserve.
- Add the vermouth and lemon juice to the butter mixture and simmer for one or two minutes.
- Add the lemon zest, red pepper, and chopped fresh parsley.
- Add the zucchini and sauté for an additional two minutes until the zoodles are slightly tender and covered with the sauce.
- Mix the shrimp with the noodles and serve with the grated Parmesan cheese.

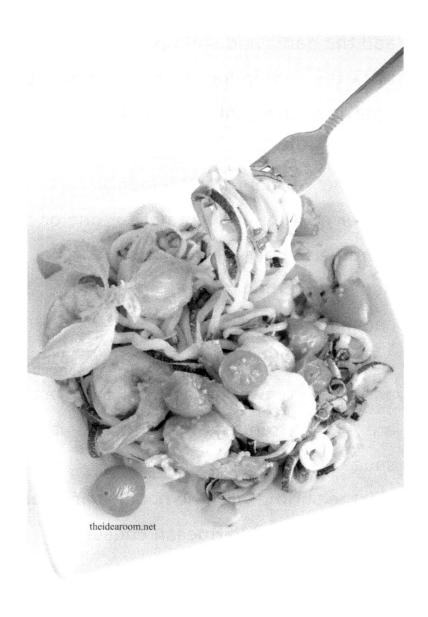

Salmon piccata with lemon sauce

Ingredients

- 4 skinless salmon fillets
- ½ teaspoon fat salt
- ½ teaspoon ground black pepper
- 3 tablespoons all-purpose flour
- 2 tablespoons olive oil
- 3 cloves garlic, minced
- ¼ cup dry white wine
- Juice of 2 lemons and slices to decorate
- 2 tablespoons capers
- 2 tablespoons chopped fresh parsley
- 2 teaspoons unsalted butter

Direction

- Gather all the ingredients of the salmon piccata.
- Sprinkle the salmon and butter with flour. Shake the excess and cook the salmon

fillets in a large pan with hot oil for two minutes, until they are browned on both sides.
- Reduce heat to medium and add chopped garlic cloves; Continue cooking for a minute.
- Add the drained lemon juice, wine, chopped fresh parsley and capers; Cook over medium-low heat until the fish is well cooked, 5 to 6 minutes. Remove the pan from the heat.
- Add the butter; Stir until it melts, about 30 seconds.
- Serve the salmon piccata with lemon sauce and decorate with the slices.

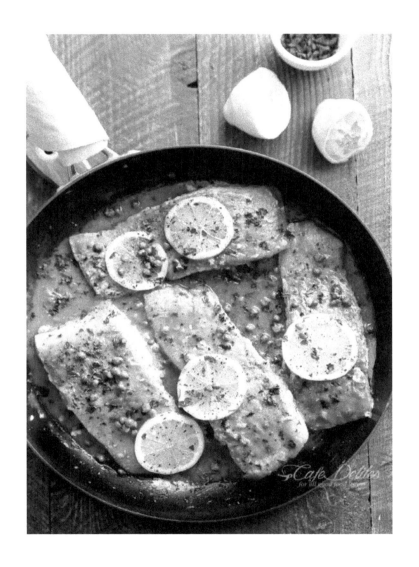

Avocado and fish cake

Ingredients

- Round puff pastry
- 3 avocados
- 125g smoked salmon
- 100ml evaporated milk
- Juice of half a lemon
- Get fat
- Garlic powder
- Fresh coriander
- Salt and ground black pepper

Direction

- Preheat the oven to 200 ° C.
- Spread the puff pastry sheet on a tray greased with oil or butter and paint it with a beaten egg.

- Place a sheet of aluminum foil over it and on this chickpeas or beans and bake for 12 minutes or until golden brown. Let it cool.
- Peel two avocados and remove the stone with a knife stroke. Remove the pulp with the help of a spoon and place it in a bowl with the evaporated milk and lemon juice.
- Mix until a homogeneous preparation.
- Add salt, garlic powder, and ground black pepper.
- Spread the avocado cream over the puff pastry, once cold.
- Peel the remaining avocado and remove the corozo. Cut it into thin strips and put them around the cake.
- Crumble the smoked salmon and put it in the center.
- Finally, decorate the avocado and fish pie with fat salt and coriander leaves.

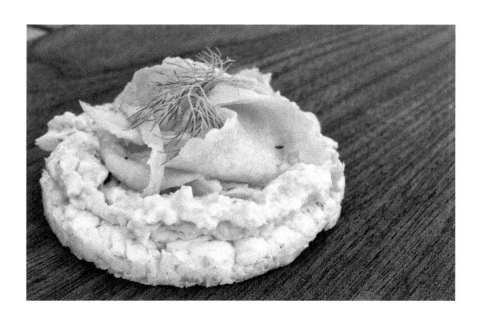

Classic French toast

Ingredients

- 6 large eggs
- 1 1/2 cups heavy cream, half and half or milk
- 2 tablespoons pure vanilla extract
- 1/2 teaspoon cinnamon
- Groundnut slicing
- Pinch of salt
- 6 slices (1-inch) bread, preferably one day
- 4 tablespoons non-alcoholic butter
- 4 tablespoons vegetable oil
- Pure maple syrup for serving (optional)

Instructions

- Mix together eggs, cream, vanilla, cinnamon, nutmeg and salt in a medium bowl; set aside.
- Put the bread in a shallow pan large enough to hold a piece of bread in one layer. Pour egg mixture on bread; soak for 10 minutes. Turn Affiliates; Simmer until simmering, about 10 minutes more.

- Preheat the oven to 250 degrees. Place a retainer on a baking sheet and set it aside. Heat 2 tablespoons oil and 2 tablespoons vegetable oil in a pan over medium heat. Cut half of the bread slices until golden brown, 2 to 3 minutes per side. Transfer to tel; place it in the oven while cooking the remaining bread. Wipe the pan and repeat with remaining butter, butter and bread. Store in the oven until ready to serve. Serve warm with pure maple syrup if desired.

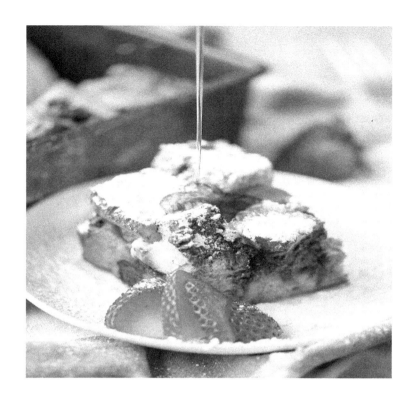

Ham 'n' Egg Sandwich

The French-speaking egg, cheese and ham sandwich is known as the Croque Madame Sandwich. For those days when the clock does not seem to slow down and the time we have seems to run out, this is a very fast recipe.

Ingredients:

- 2 eggs Aido's house.
- 4 slices of bread or baguette.
- 50 g of butter.
- 4 large slices of cheese.
- 2 large slices of ham.
- 2 lettuce leaves.
- Salt, pepper, and herbs to taste.

Preparation:

- Spread the butter on the bread and brown in a dry skillet.
- Remove 2 slices from the pan and place the cheese slices and let it melt a little.
- Place the ham over the cheese and top with a lettuce leaf.
- Put another slice of cheese and top with bread.

- Cover the pan and brown the sandwich for 30 seconds.
- Fry the egg using a mold seasoning with salt and pepper to the desired point.

Nutrition Facts

543 calories, 31 g fat (14 g saturated fat), 298 mg cholesterol, 1644 mg sodium, 33 g carbohydrate, 32 g protein.

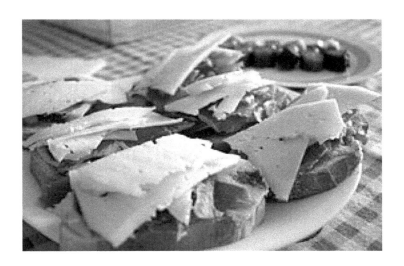

Bagel Recipe with Egg and Ham

The egg and ham bagel is a breakfast recipe you'll love. Especially if you wake up late during the weekend, you can prepare this bagel recipe and have a brunch accompanied by a shake.

Ingredients:
- 1 unit of bagel
- 2 slices of ham
- 1 slice of cheese
- 1 unit of egg
- 1 pinch of salt
- 1 handful of arugula
- 1 teaspoon mustard
- 1 tablespoon mayonnaise

Steps to make this recipe:
- To start making this recipe prepare all the ingredients. Remember that you can modify the extras as you like.
- First, let's make the poached egg. To do this put the egg in cling film, put some salt and close tightly as shown in the picture, then bake in boiling water for 8 minutes.

- Aside, make the sauce by adding light mayonnaise and mustard. If you want you can also add some English sauce.
- Lightly toast the bagel, and stuff it with the arugula leaves and in the other slice put the sauce. Then place the ham and cheese on the arugula leaves. If you prefer the melted cheese, pass the ham and cheese lightly on the grill.
- Finally, lay the poached egg and enjoy! This recipe can also be served with some Dutch sauce. Moreover, it is perfect to accompany for example a banana and raspberry smoothie.

Nutritional information

1 sandwich: 427 calories, 21g fat (11g saturated fat), 56mg cholesterol, 791mg sodium, 41g carbohydrates (5g sugars, 4g fiber), 20g protein.

French Toast with Apple and Raisins

Ingredients

- raw egg 1 pcs
- skimmed milk 1 cup
- Sweetener 1 CS
- Clove, ground 1 pinch (s)
- french toast bread 1 pcs big ones)
- apple without shell 1 pcs stings
- seedless white raisins ¼ cups
- light margarine 1 CS, melted
- cinnamon powder 1 pinch (s)

Instructions

- Grease a medium refractory pan with spray oil and set aside. Apart, beat the egg lightly and add the milk, sweetener, and cloves, combining well. Add the bread cubes, apples and raisins, mixing lightly. Set aside until the bread absorbs all the liquid.
- In a bowl, combine margarine and cinnamon. Spread the bread with the apple in the reserved form. Cover with cinnamon mixture. Bake in a

moderately preheated oven (180 ° C) for 30 minutes or until golden brown.

Meatloaf With Sweet Potato

INGREDIENTS

Meatloaf:

- 800 g of ground beef (duckling or rump)
- 1 envelope of onion cream
- 2 eggs
- 3 cloves garlic, minced
- 1 onion, finely chopped
- 1/2 cup minced green smell
- salt to taste

Filling:

- 2 chopped seedless tomatoes
- 1 chopped onion
- 1 large grated carrot
- Salt and pepper to taste
- catupiry (curd or grated mozzarella)

Other Ingredients:

- 12 to 15 bacon slices
- 5 sweet potatoes cut in 4 (pre-steamed)
- 3 thick sliced onions
- olive oil

PREPARATION

Filling:

- Mix tomatoes, onions, carrots, salt and pepper in a bowl. Reserve.

Meatloaf:

- In another bowl, mix all ingredients of the meatloaf well.
- With your hands, open the mixture on top of a plastic wrap or open plastic bag (this will make it easier to roll up).
- Spread the filling.
- Put the cheese of your choice (catupiry, curd or mozzarella).
- Close the roll, like a roll, and top with the bacon slices.
- In a baking dish, spread a drizzle of olive oil and make a layer with the onions in slices. Place the meatloaf over it.
- On the sides, add the remaining onions and sweet potatoes.
- Bake (at 220ºC) for about 30 minutes until well browned.

Additional Information

- Tips & Warnings Instead of sweet potatoes, use common potatoes. The filling can be modified according to your creativity. Add black olives, palm hearts or grated cabbage, for example. The filling should be very dry so as not to drop water when closing and baking the roll. Therefore use tomatoes without the seed. If necessary, close the ends of the roll with barbecue sticks. But remember to take them out when serving. To accompany, green salad and white rice. The onion cream and bacon already have enough salt. Be careful when adding more.

Cracker Barrel Meatloaf

Material

Meatloaf ingredients

- 1 1/2 lb ground chuck
- 2 eggs
- 1 cup of crushed litz cracker
- 1/4 cup milk
- 1/2 cup finely chopped white onion
- Finely chopped blue peppers 1/4 cup
- 14.1 oz canned tomato-can drain
- 1 tsp salt
- Black tea pepper 1/4 teaspoon

Meatloaf glaze

- 1/2 cup ketchup
- 2 tablespoons brown sugar
- 1 tsp yellow mustard
- 1 tsp Worcester sauce

INSTRUCTIONS

Meatloaf Glaze Preparation

- Ketchup, brown sugar, mustard, and Worcestershire sauce are combined in a small bowl.

Meatloaf Preparation

- Preheat oven to 350 degrees F. For easy removal if needed line a baking sheet with parchment paper or aluminum foil.
- Beat the eggs well in a large bowl, then add the crumbs of cracker, onion, green pepper, milk, salt, diced tomatoes drained, and pepper. Play well with each other.
- Add beef to the ground and blend well. Shape the meatloaf mixture into a loaf onto the prepared pan.
- Bake and spread over the meatloaf for 30 minutes. Bake for another 30 minutes or until 160 ° F is in the middle.
- Let rest for 5-10 minutes, then slice and serve.

Nutrition

Calories: 253kcal | Carbohydrates: 12g | Protein: 14g | Fat: 16g | Saturated Fat: 6g | Cholesterol: 82mg | Sodium: 472mg | Potassium: 347mg | Fiber: 1g | Sugar: 7g | | Calcium: 51mg | Iron: 2mg

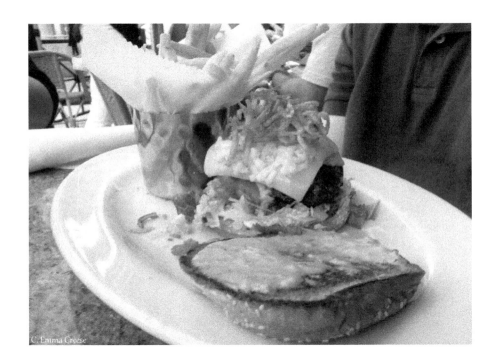

Senate bean soup with ham

What do you need

- 1 pound
- marine beans (or large northern beans, dried, washed and drained)
- 1 bone of meaty ham (or 2 smoked hocks)
- 3 medium potatoes (cooked and mashed)
- 1 1/2 cups of onion (chopped)
- 1 1/2 cups of celery (chopped)
- 2 tablespoons of parsley (fresh, chopped)
- 2 large
- cloves garlic (minced)
- Salt to taste
- Black pepper to taste

How to do it

- Cover the beans with water and cook for 2 minutes. Remove from heat, cover and allow 1 to 2 hours to stand.
- Place the colander on a bowl and pour the liquid from the beans. Measure and add enough water or unsalted vegetable soup to make 2 liters. Pour

- the liquid into the beans and add the ham bone or ham hook, onions, celery and garlic.
- Bring to a boil the beans. Reduce heat to a minimum, cover the pan and cook for about 2 hours, or until very tender beans.
- Attach the mashed potatoes, carrots, celery, parsley and garlic and cook for another hour. Cut the bone or hocks from the ham and cut from the bones the meat. Cut the meat and put it back in the soup.
- Season with salt and pepper.

Tips

- Bring the soup to a potluck or party. Transfer the cooked hot soup to a slow cooker and put it on low to serve.

Nutritional guidelines

- calories   274
- Totally fat   1 g
- Saturated fats   0 g
- Unsaturated fats 0 g
- Cholesterol 2 mg

- Sodium   109 mg
- carbohydrates   52 g
- Dietary fiber   13 g
- Protein   15 g

Chick fil A sandwich

Material

Marinade

- 2 cups of water
- 2 cube chicken bouillon
- 1/4 teaspoon of seasoned salt

Bread crumbs

- 1 cup general purpose flour
- 1 1/2 cup finely ground salty cracker crumbs
- 2 teaspoon powdered sugar
- 1/4 teaspoon paprika

Ingredients for sandwiches

- 4 hamburger buns
- 8 dill pickles
- 2 tablespoons butter
- You can use peanut oil vegetable oil for frying

Instructions

Chicken marinade procedure

- Add cold water to the bowl, add 1/4 teaspoon of seasoned salt and dissolve the bouillon cube in the mixture. Put chicken breasts in water, mix, cover, and refrigerate for 12 hours or the next day.

Chicken dough steps

- Pour the chicken marinade and discard it. It cannot be used again.
- In a small bowl, mix universal flour, crackers, powdered sugar and paprika. Shuffle to combine.
- Shake off excess marinade and sprinkle flour on chicken.
- Place the beaten chicken breasts on a wire rack and leave for a few minutes.

Cooking chicken

- Heat the oil to 350 degrees in a tempura pan or large pan. If you are using a large pot, add enough oil so that the oil is 4 inches deep.
- Cook the chicken for 7-8 minutes or until the chicken turns brown and the internal temperature

reaches 165 ° C. Drain the chicken into a clean wire rack.

Collect sandwiches

- Melt the butter and clean with a burger roll.
- Place one chicken sandwich on each bottom of the hamburger.
- Pickles of two dill, and top bread.

Nutrition

Calories: 781kcal | Carbohydrates: 69g | Protein: 35g | Fat: 40g | Saturated Fat: 10g | Cholesterol: 87mg | Sodium: 1956mg | Potassium: 667mg | Fiber: 4g | Sugar: 6g | Vitamin A: 508IU | Vitamin C: 3mg | Calcium: 149mg | Iron: 5mg

CPSIA information can be obtained
at www.ICGtesting.com
Printed in the USA
LVHW021022180121
676773LV00003B/279